represents a urinal, which was the most important instrument of the physician up to the 18th century.

Checking the colour, smell, and taste of the urine in the glass, the doctor was able to make a diagnosis. St. Damian, patron saint of the apothecaries, too, has a characteristic vessel: in his right hand, he holds a kind of a small mortar for the preparation of ointments and in his left a spatula, ready to mix the ingredients.

The twin saints reflect the proximity of the two professions. Doctors had already been practicing their profession in the period of Classical antiquity, whereas first quotations of apothecaries appear only in medieval sources. Those are wordings of law such as the epochal body of laws of the famous German Emperor Frederic II. (1194–1250) of the Kingdom of Sicily (Liber Augustalis 1231/1240), in which he laid down stipulations about the outline of the professions of doctors and apothecaries. However, it still took some time until apothecary shops opened hereabouts as well. We find them in the prospering medieval towns since the 13th/14th century.

Until then, medical care had mostly been practiced in monasteries, where also the antique medical and pharmaceutical knowledge was kept. As another fo-

▲ *Left: St. Cosmas, right: St. Damian, Switzerland, 18th century.*

cus of the collection, the German Museum of Pharmacy reflects those early roots of pharmacy with a multitude of former monastic equipment in the exhibition.

An **apothecary cupboard,** dating from the period about 1740, comes from the monastery of the Discalded Carmelites at Schongau in Bavaria. Its compartment doors have pictures of several monasteries of the order in Bavaria. From the left: the monasteries in Regensburg and Augsburg, the mother monastery in Munich and the monastery in Urfahrn (today Reisach, Inn). Absent is a depiction of the Schongau monastery, which must have been on the now missing fifth compartment at the right hand side of the cupboard. On the picture of the Munich monastery, there is a large tree growing out of the building, its branches reaching to the left and right over the other monasteries. The tree and its branches symbolize the biblical Tree of Knowledge and the foundation of the younger monasteries, originating from the principal monastery in Munich. The lower doors of the cupboard have two kinds of decoration. On the left side, there is a 19th century adornment (aloe). The others show the restored original decoration. Finally, there is also a very rare treasure inside the cupboard: its original equipment with more than 180 glass vessels, all filled with the original medical ingredients of the 18th century.

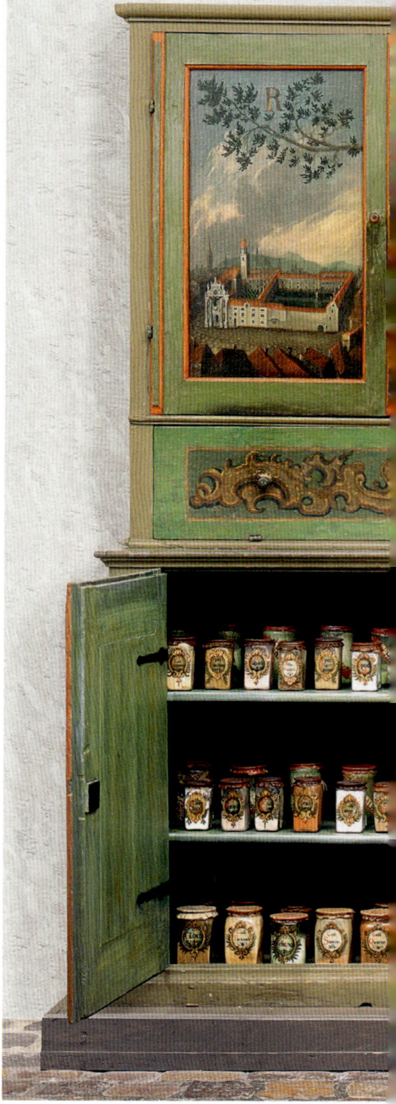

▶ *Cupboard for medicine, monastery of Schongau, about 1740.*

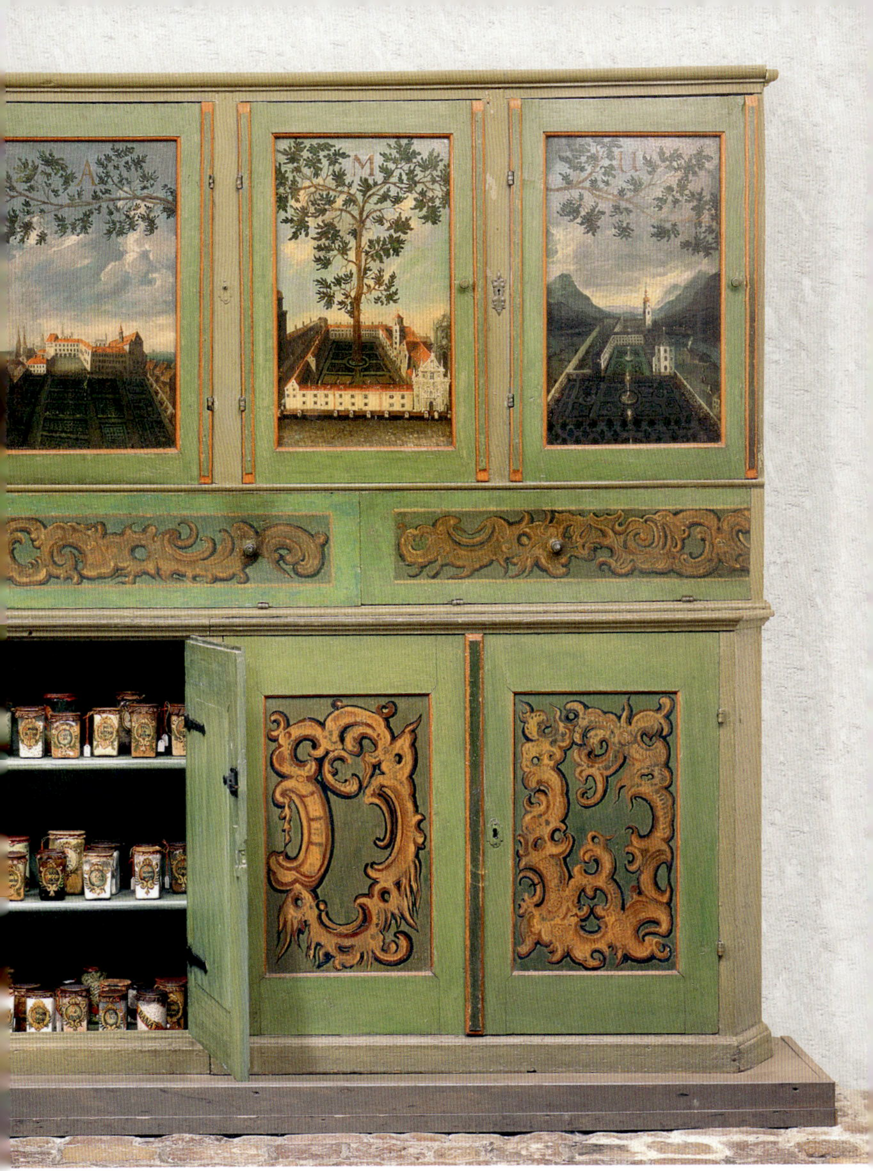
A
M
U

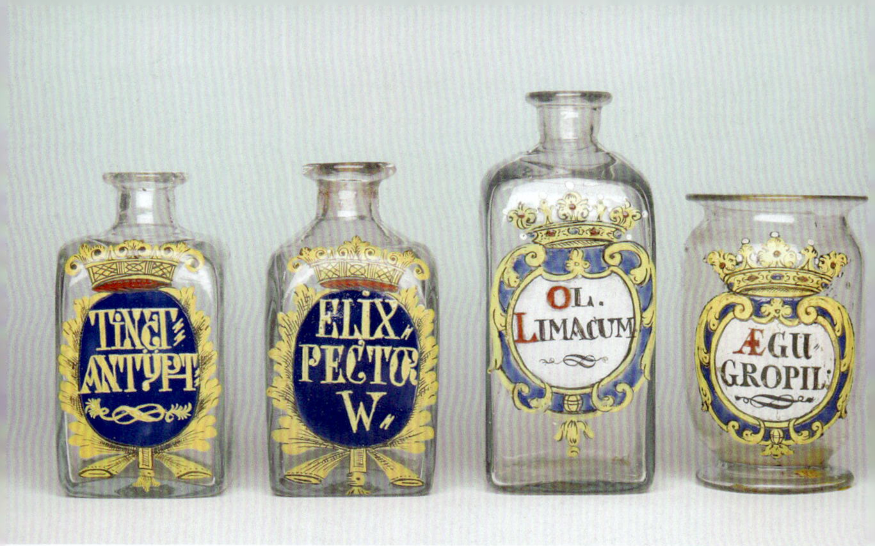

Room 2 – Historical Survey

Room 2 offers an outline of medicine from the period of Classical antiquity to the 21st century. European medicine up to the 18th century had drawn its knowledge from several sources, most importantly from the medical knowledge of the Antiquity and its reception through the Byzantine Empire; from Persia and the Arabic-Islamic cultural room, as well as from indigenous traditions reflected especially in the monastic medicine. The texts are illustrated by exhibits such as innovations, classics of the age, and similar. One display case, for example, contains Roman unguentaria, or tears vessels, (1st century BC), Persian ceramics of the 14th century, the oldest dated wooden pharmaceutical vessels of the German speaking area (1607/08 AD), an old specimen of the standardized medical weight from Nuremberg (introduced in 1555 AD), and the first official pharmacopoeia (Valerius Cordus 1546 AD). A multifunctional steam driven distillation apparatus stands for the influence of industrialization in the chemist's shop.

▲ *Enamel painted glass vessels, 18th century.*

The baroque "officina" (Lat. for workshop) of the Benedictine monastery in Schwarzach (Baden/Rheinmünster, about 1724 AD) dominates the center of the room. It is painted in light green with a subtle accentuation in gold. On the oaken top of the preparation table, the antique god of healing, Aesculapius, and his daughter Hygieia keep an eye on the preparation of the medicine. They hold

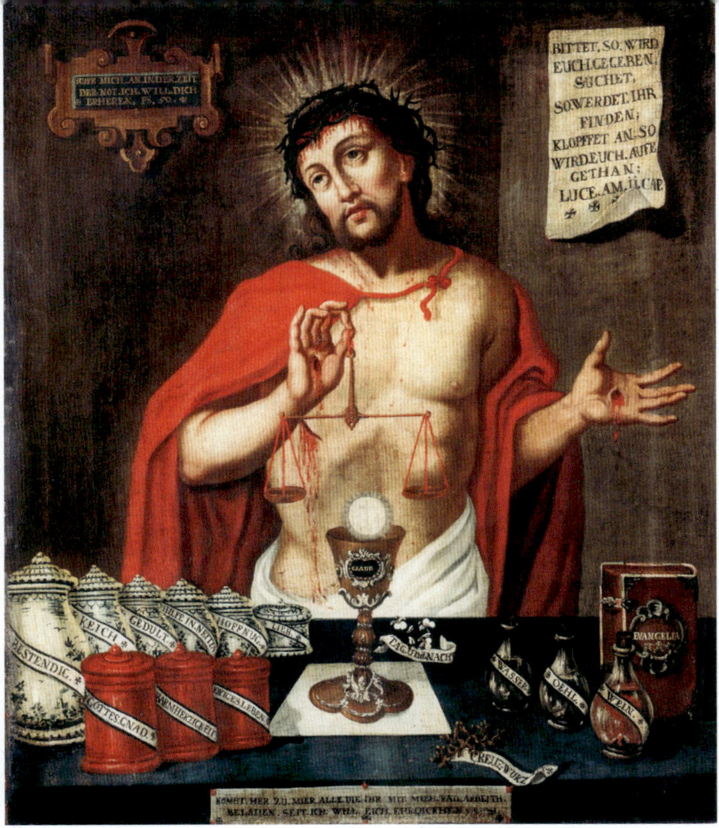

their specific symbol in their hands, a snake wound around a staff. The shelves contain a part of the famous and worldwide largest collection of enamel painted glass vessels, originating mainly from central Germany of the 18th century.

Opposite the officina, a group of exhibits treats the topic of "faith and healing". Several paintings show the popular motive of Christ preparing medicine at a pharmacy. It symbolizes the conviction that real healing (of the soul) is only possible through God. Therefore, the vessels do not contain pharmaceutical ingredients, but Christian virtues (such as mercy). The prescription book is the Bible, and the scale does not weigh medical ingredients but the souls at the Day of the

▲ ***Christ in a pharmacist's shop, Munich, 2nd half of the 18th century.***

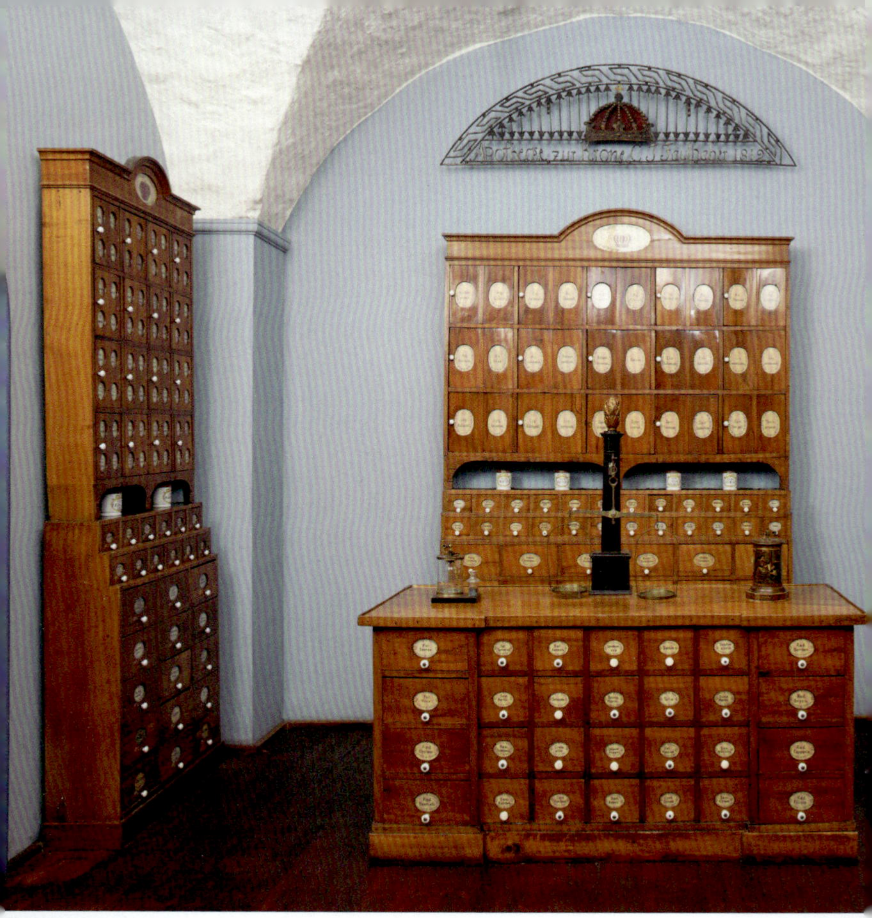

Last Judgement. A collection of religious folk art exhibits (amulets, votive offerings from the 17th–19th centuries) and several statues of saints (St. Sebastian and St. Roche, patron saints of the Black Death, St. Mary Magdalene, patroness of the apothecaries) illustrate the width of this topic.

▲ *Crown Pharmacy Ulm, furniture of about 1812–1814.*

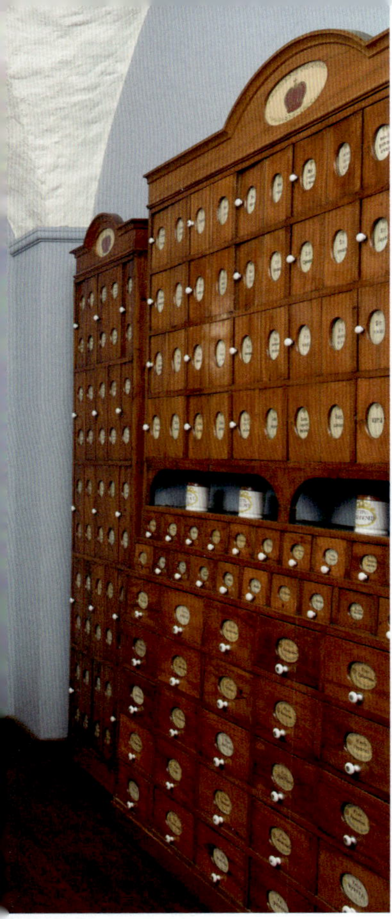

Rooms 3 and 4 – Children's Pharmacy and Pharmacy in the Biedermeier Style

Room 3 is an important site for the frequent educational activities of the museum. Here children can work as little chemists to their heart's content.

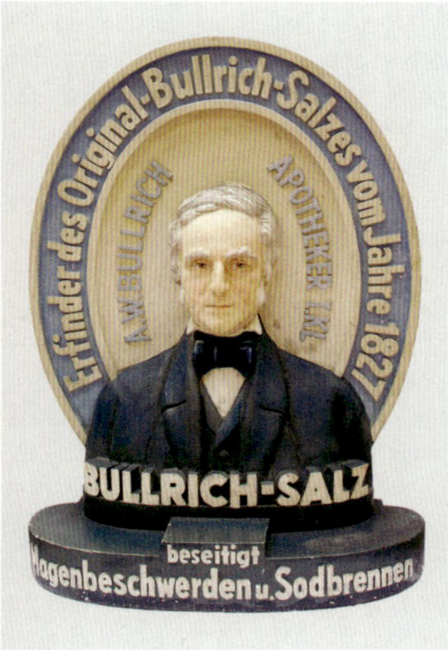

Room 4 displays additional interesting authentic furnishings. The light blue paint of the walls reproduces the original wall colour of the old **Crown Pharmacy at Ulm** ("Apotheke zur Krone", about 1812–14), perfectly framing the warm cherrywood furniture. The shelfsystem containing the vessels has been untypically designed as a closed cupboard. The artistic sense and long experience of the owner of the drugstore, Christoph Jacob Faulhaber (1772–1842), was an important influence on the design: doors sheltered the medicine from light and vermin.

▲ *The chemist August Wilhelm Bullrich advertised the Bullrichsalt, named after him, "in person", in the shopwindow of the drugstore. Half figure, hard plastic, about 1950.*

Double labelling, outside on the doors and inside on the containers, prevented mistakes. But there was also an eminent disadvantage: this kind of closed instead of open shelving soon run in conflict with the official regulations and in 1898 an inspection complained of this violation of the law. The officina was decommissioned and moved to the Town Museum of Ulm. After the destruction of Ulm's Moor's Pharmacy in World War II, the old furnishings of the Crown Pharmacy were recommissioned and served on up to demands for quite a time. Only when the Moor's Pharmacy had moved to a new residence in 1959 including new, modern furnishings, the valuable old cupboards found their final location in the German Museum of Pharmacy.

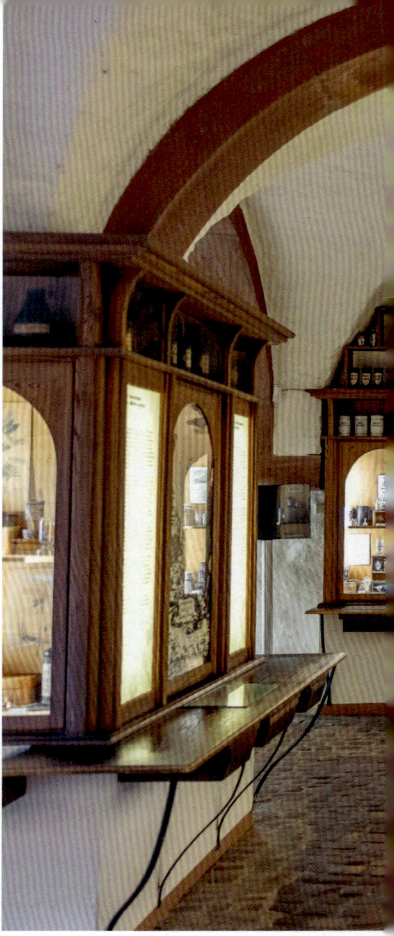

Room 5 – The Medicament

The German Museum of Pharmacy owns the worldwide largest stock of the "materia medica" of the 17th–20th centuries. The Latin term "materia medica" stands for the whole of all raw materials, which were either used as medicaments themselves, or which were processed into medicaments. In the pharmaceutical terminology, all raw materials with medical use are described as "drugs" (derived from "dry"). The range of medicaments included plant (vegetabilia), animal (animalia) and mineral drugs (mineralia). The realm of plants was the oldest and for a long time most used source for extraction of pharmaceutical substances (e.g. leaves, blooms, seeds, roots, or secretions). About 10–20 % of the drugs come from the realm of animals. Grease was used as a base for ointments and the horn of the legendary unicorn – which in reality was the tooth of the narwhal – was held in high esteem because of its supposed antitoxic effects. Already since

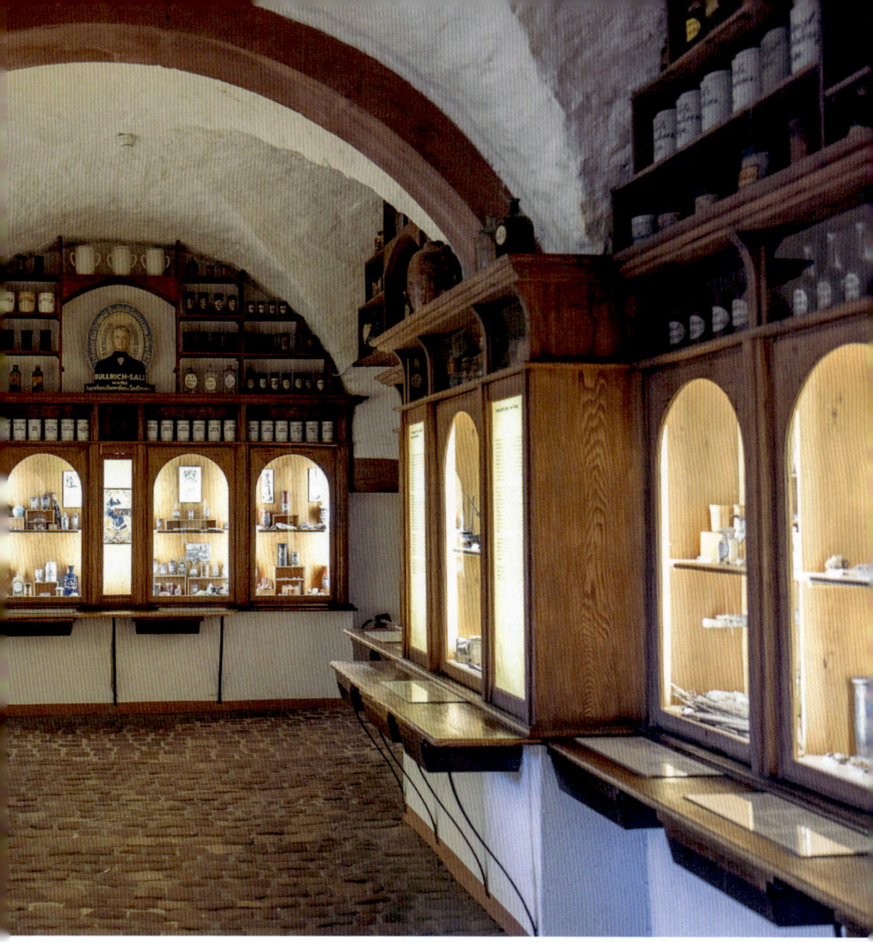

Classical antiquity, stones, metals, and earths have been counted to the realm of minerals, and they have acquired an ever increasing interest since the age of **Paracelsus (1493/94–1541).**

The 28 display cases in room 5 present more than a thousand raw materials, systematically arranged according either to active agents or to indications. Plant or animal drawings and medical vessels of the 17th–19th centuries accompany

▲ *View into the collection of medicaments.*

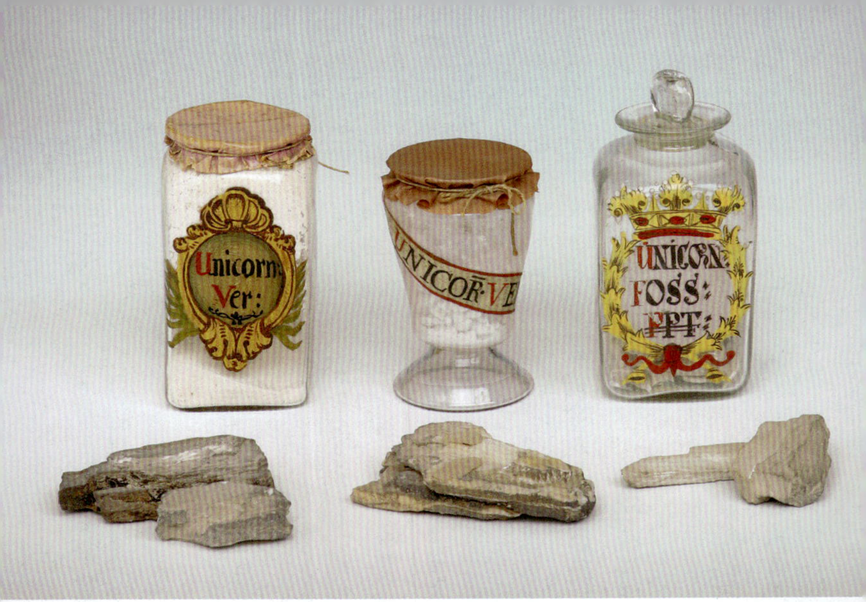

▲ *Glass vessels for the "real" unicorn (tooth of the narwhal), on the right for fossil unicorn (tooth of the mammoth), Germany, 18th century.*

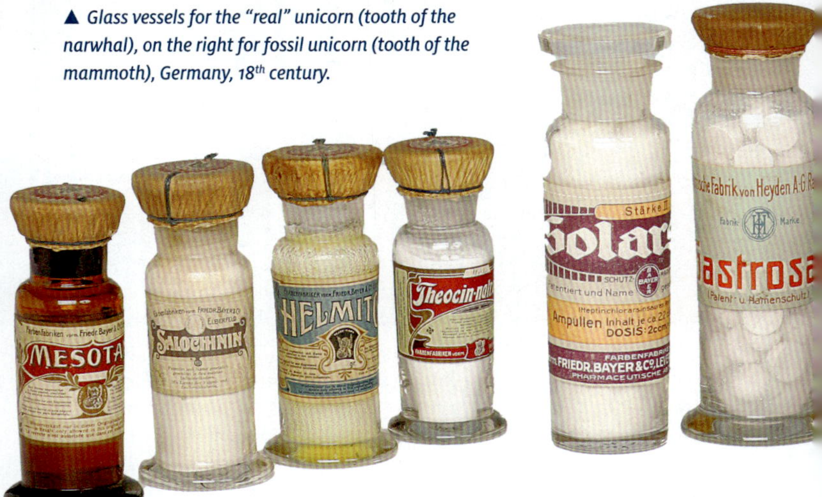

▲ *Early manufactured medicaments, 1910/30.*

them. There are sage and St. John's wort, as well as now obsolete medicaments like the antipyretic bark of the cinchona tree (used against malaria since the 17th century). They are joined by materials such as tea, cocoa and spices, which had been first introduced in Europe as medicaments but soon have turned into consumer goods. In addition, there are strange preparations of the "unicorn", of mummy powder, and human grease. A whole showcase is dedicated to the **"Queen of the medicaments",** the "theriac". This jam-like mixture of dark colour that had first been mixed out of 60 ingredients in Classical antiquity which had increased up to 200 in the 18th century, was an indispensable classic in the range of medicaments. The

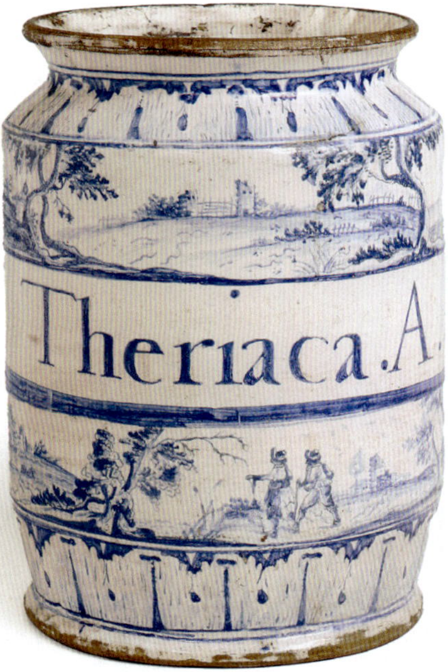

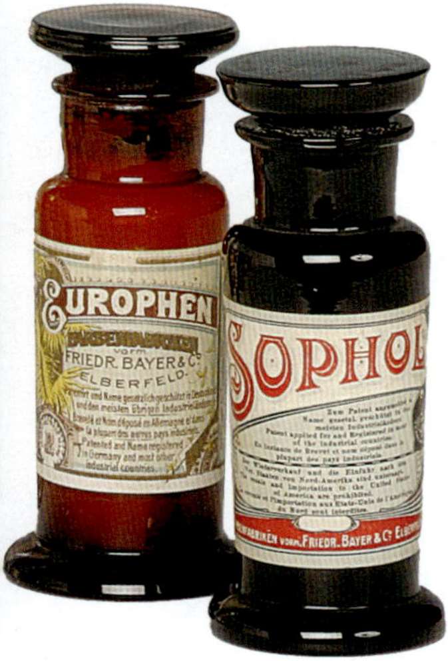

mixture, praised as a universal remedy, consisted mainly of plant components (such as black pepper, rose leaves, root of violet, liquorice, myrrh), but also of narcotics like opium, and of such animal ingredients as viper's flesh, for example.

Industrial production of medicaments, introduced in the late 19th century, is presented in the back of room 5. The most important pharmaceutical milestones of the 20th century are

▲ *A splendid jar of theriac, majolica, Talavera, about 1700.*

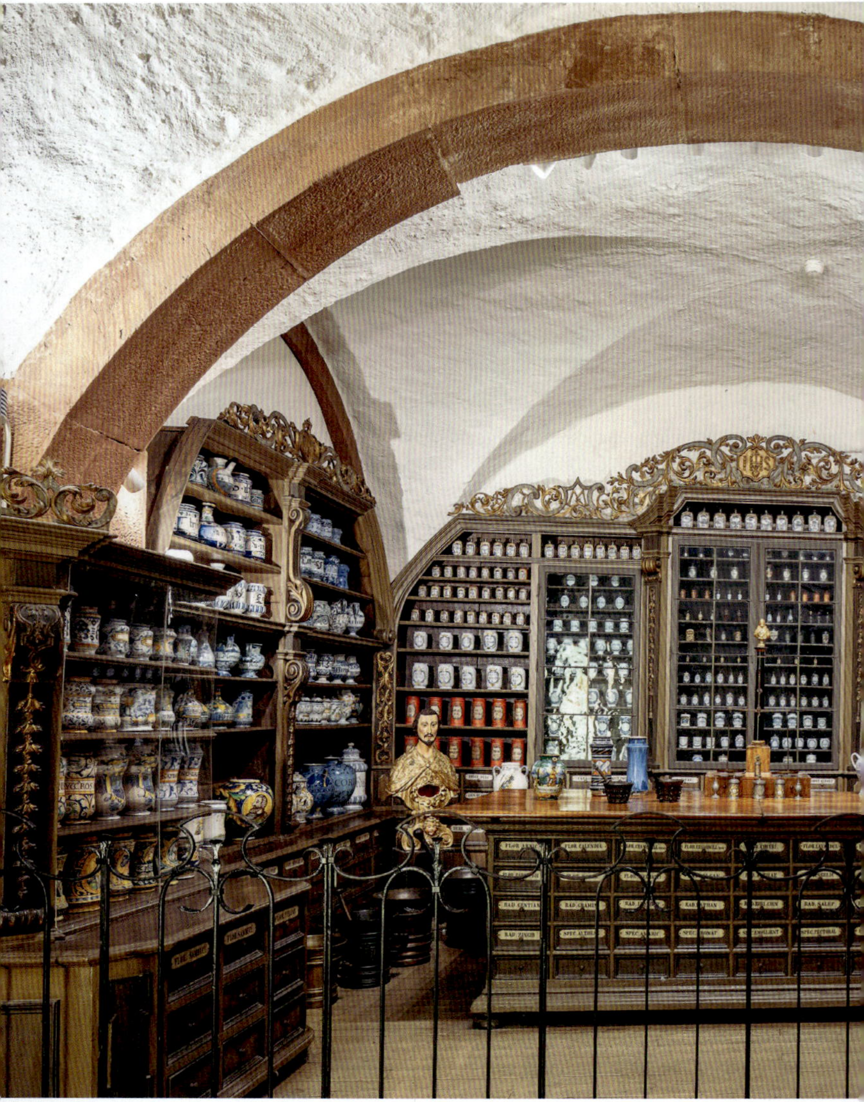
FLOR CALENDUL
RAD GENTIAN
RAD SALEP
RAD ZINGIB
SPEC PECTORAL

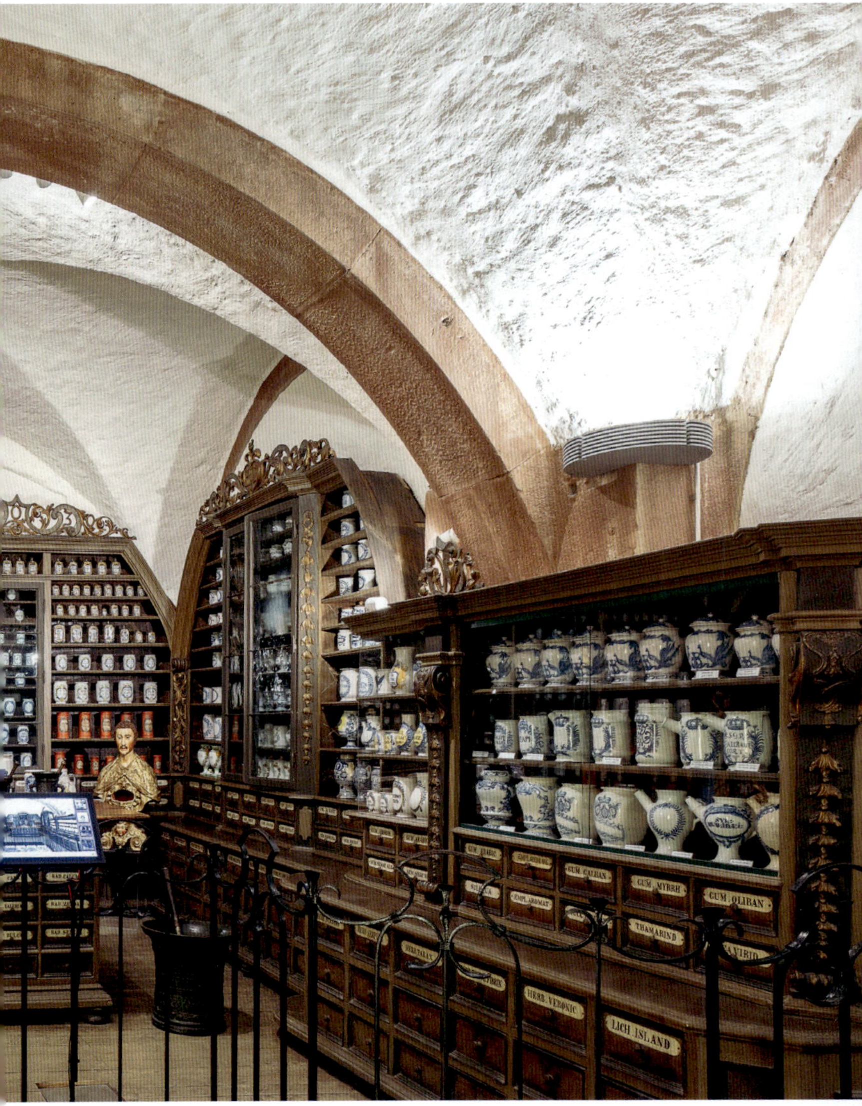

▲ *Officina of the Ursuline convent of Klagenfurt, 1730.*

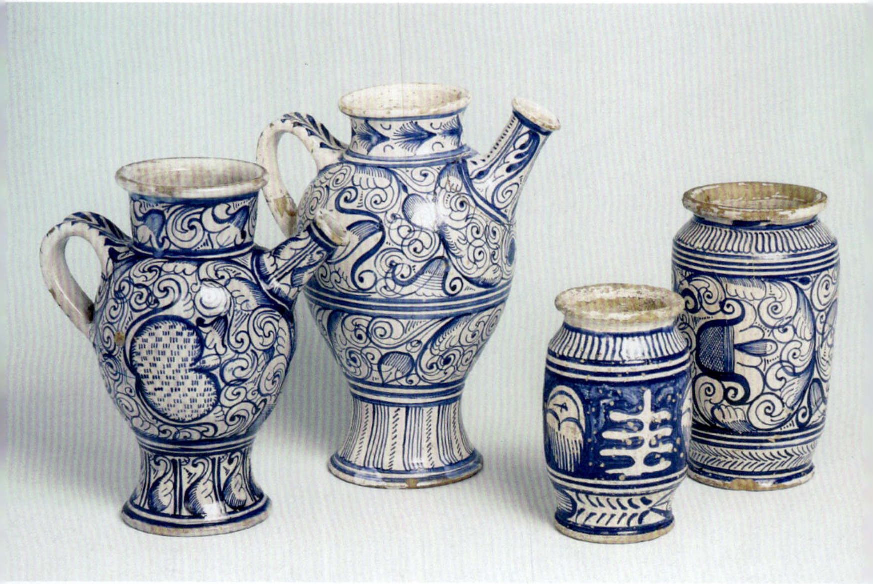

displayed here, among them aspirin (1917) and penicillin (1947). There are also rarities, such as the first manufactured medicaments of the time around 1900.

Room 6 – The Officina

The Latin term "officina" means workshop. This is where medicaments had been prepared. A small stock of simple raw materials (simplicia) as well as mixed preparations (composita) had been kept in vessels and drawers. On the worktable, the pharmacist prepared the medicament following the doctor's prescription. In the old days, the client had only been allowed to look into the room through a window. Until the $18^{th}/19^{th}$ century, this was the usual way of communication with the pharmacist. Only later, access to the officina has gradually been granted to the client.

▲ *Faience vessels, Arnstadt, 17th century.*

CONVENT OF THE URSULINES, KLAGENFURT

In the convent, medicaments for the needs of both the nuns and of the inhabitants of the surrounding villages were prepared. The apothecaries of neighbouring towns were often angry about the too

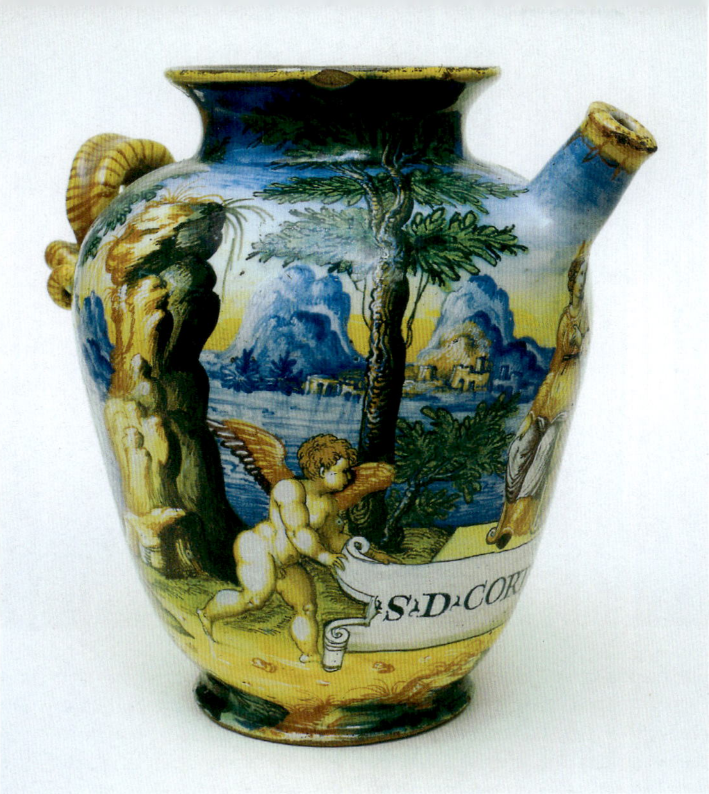

small charges demanded for the medicine at the convent's door. The officina of the Ursulines appears magnificently: gilded plant arabesques crown the shelves; in the center, there is the monogram of Christ, "IHS", and to the right and left, two pairs of numbers are entwined within the arabesques. They give the date of its foundation 1730. The mighty size of the preparation table is emphasized by its large walnut top, which was added in the 19th century. The present colour scheme dates from this time as well. According to a restoration examination, the furniture was originally colourful: green and red with gold accentuations, and white-red marbled base mouldings.

The shelves accommodate a **splendid majolica and faience collection:** on the left, colourful pieces of Italian ma-

▲ *Syrup jar from the famous Fontana workshop at Urbino, 1542/1571.*

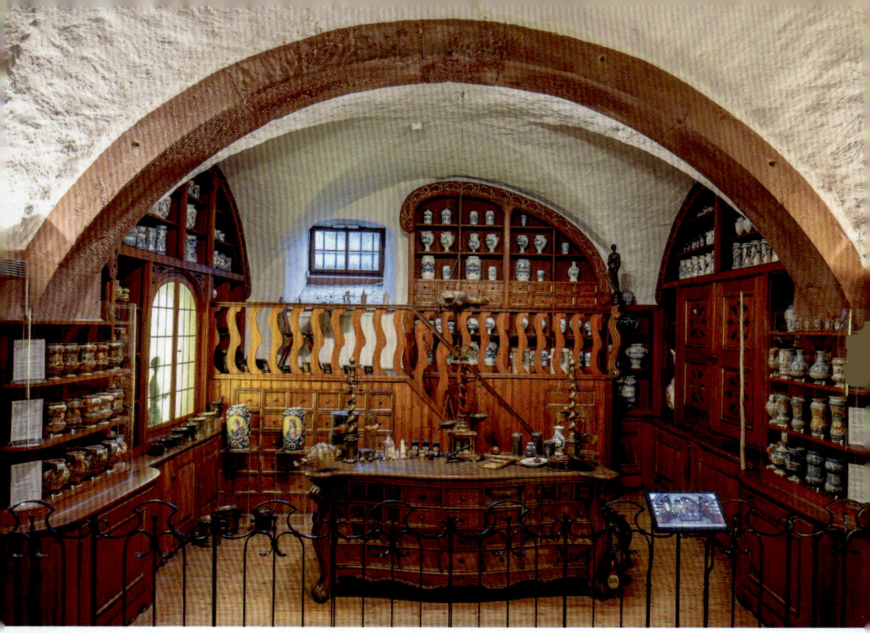

jolica of the 15th–17th centuries (e.g. from Faenza, Savona, Venice), on the right, products of German manufactories of the 18th century. They are gleaming white with filigreed cartouches in blue, showing garlands of leaves (e.g. from Hanau, Nuremberg, Durlach). Early faiences of Arnstadt (17th century) are the other highlight.

COURT PHARMACY, BAMBERG

Baroque furnishings of the Court Pharmacy in Bamberg, among them a preparation table from the time about 1730/40, constitute a vivid display. This public pharmacist's shop of the 18th century has been put up as a contrast to the clerical furnishings to the right. The client and the apothecary could communicate through a window, which allowed a view into the officina from outside. This explains why the pharmacist attached great value to its arrangement: long rows of splendid vessels, diverse tools, and very often a centrally positioned eyecatcher. A viewer, who rarely crossed the confines of his town, could easily gain an impression of an exotic, strange, and mysterious world, seeing a fine tooth of the narwhal or a stuffed crocodile.

▲ *Furniture of the Court Pharmacy in Bamberg, about 1730/40.*

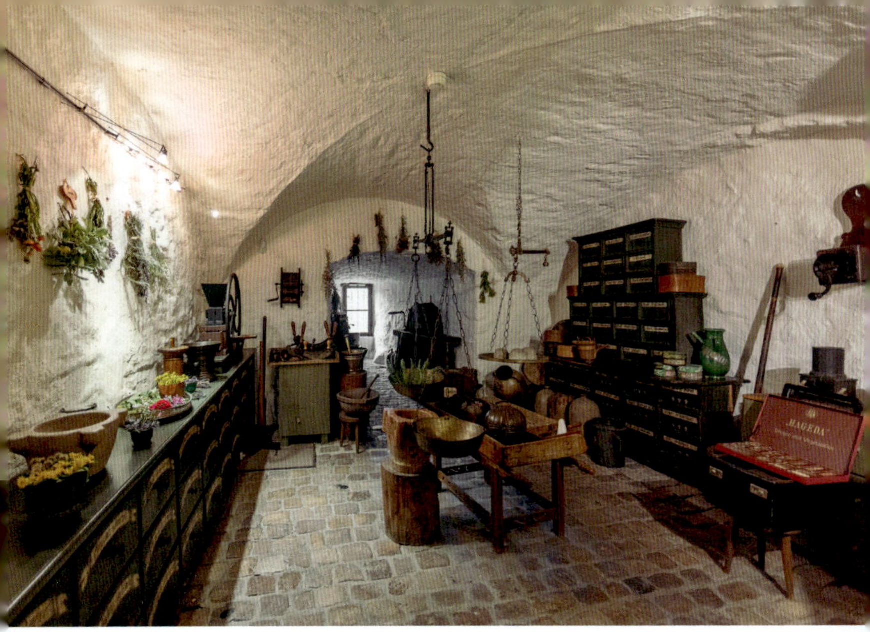

Room 7 – The Store Room

A special room, often situated in the attic of the pharmacy, served for dry storage of the **pharmaceutical material and herbs.** Since the 19th century, more and more chemicals had been stored here in addition to plants and other raw materials. Typical storage equipment consisted of large containers (pitchers, wicker bottles), drying racks, as well as simple high shelves with roomy drawers. One of the oldest pieces of furniture of the museum's collection is the **cupboard with drawers** from the **Town Pharmacy of Mosbach** (17th century). The three lower rows of drawers deserve a special notice: each drawer carries three white crosses. This was meant to be a precaution measure, as only strongly effective, even dangerous drugs were stored there, such as leaves of digitalis (foxglove, used for cardiac tonics). Diverse tools from the 17th–19th centuries illustrate the multiple steps during the processing of raw materials. There are valuable mortars but also simple chopping knives, as well as wooden cutting boards, grinders and scales for the weighing of large quantities.

▲ *Store room for herbs and material, with furnishings of the Town Pharmacy Mosbach, 17th century.*

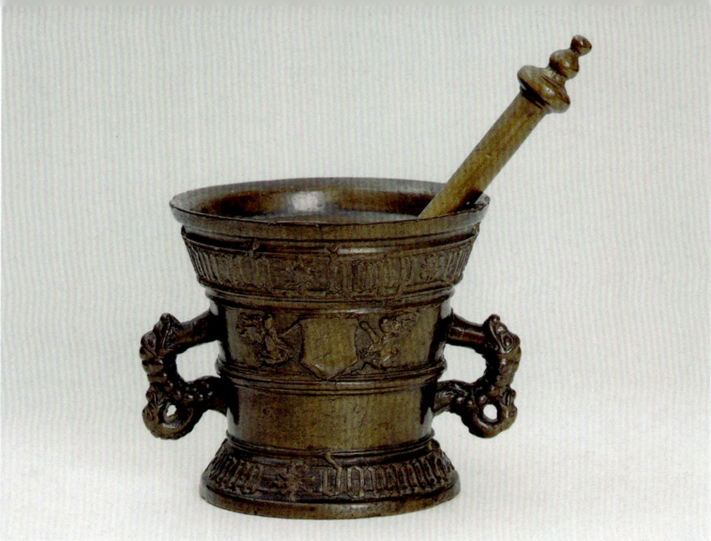

Room 8 – Emblems of Pharmacies

For centuries, an original, individual **emblem** was part of the outer appearance of each pharmacist's shop. Decorated plaques indicated the name of the shop and of its owner. Often, figures of animals, fabulous creatures or patron saints illustrated the drugstore's name. The indication 'Council' or 'Town' pharmacy referred to legal relations. In addition, there were biblical (St. Mary's Pharmacy) or regional links: Lion pharmacies are often found in territories which have lions as heraldic beasts in their princes' coat of arms (in Bavaria, for example). Eagle pharmacies are typical for Prussia, where the eagle was an omnipresent heraldic beast. Fabulous beasts like the unicorn were popular name patrons as well.

"Emblems of Pharmacies" is another main focus of the museum's collection, which includes not only some of the oldest plaques (such as the Court Pharmacy of Füssen, 1696) and many charming animal figures, but also follows the winding path of the development of the current symbol of pharmacies. Preliminary stages are illustrated through singular exhibits, such as the first unified emblem (1928) and also **"the emblem of the three spoons"** from the late twenties with its radical, modern design in the style of "The New Objectivity". It did not survive the seizure of power of the National Socialists.

▲ *Bronze mortar of the workshop Hachmann, Kleve, 1554.*

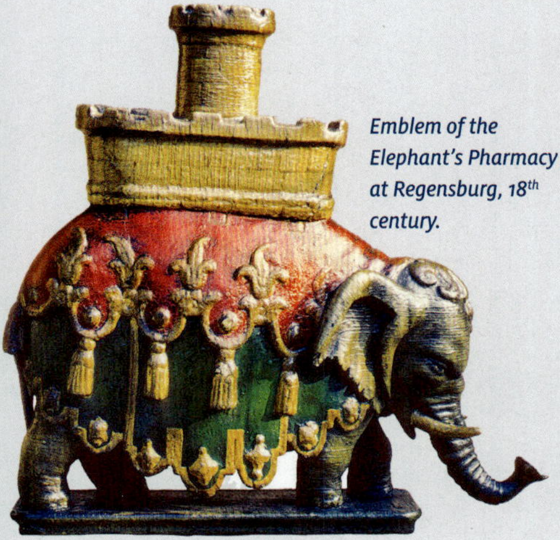

Emblem of the Elephant's Pharmacy at Regensburg, 18th century.

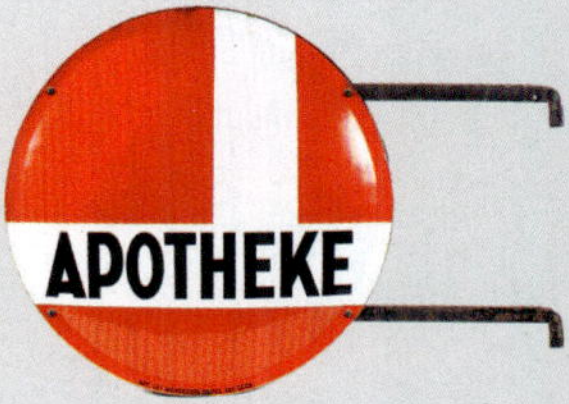

First unified emblem, 1928.

Emblem of the three spoons, about 1930.

Room 9 – Temporary Exhibition

Highlights of the museum's collection are displayed in rotation here, such as 19th century objects from the written legacy of the morphine-discoverer Friedrich-Wilhelm Sertürner (1783–1841). Exhibits from the Modern Age represent specimens of "the good form" ideal, such as the pharmaceutical vessels of the **Sicherer Pharmacy at Heilbronn:** these were designed by the famous industrial designers Wilhelm Wagenfeld (1900–1990) and Heinrich Löffelhardt (1901–1979).

Room 10 – The Laboratory

The room is situated in the impressive **"Apothecary's Tower"**, a part of the former fortifications of the Heidelberg Castle. This arrangement of the laboratory (= workroom, derived from Lat. labor) offers a look into yet another workroom of the pharmacy. Hearths were most important here, for their heat was necessary for the processing and production of many medicaments. Alchemy played a central role in the development of the laboratory equipment. Although the medieval Europe of the 12th century was becoming slowly acquainted with the Arabian alchemy, only a few of its methods and techniques had at first been used here. Not until the time after Paracelsus (1493/94–1541), during the 15th–16th centuries, we see an increasing reception

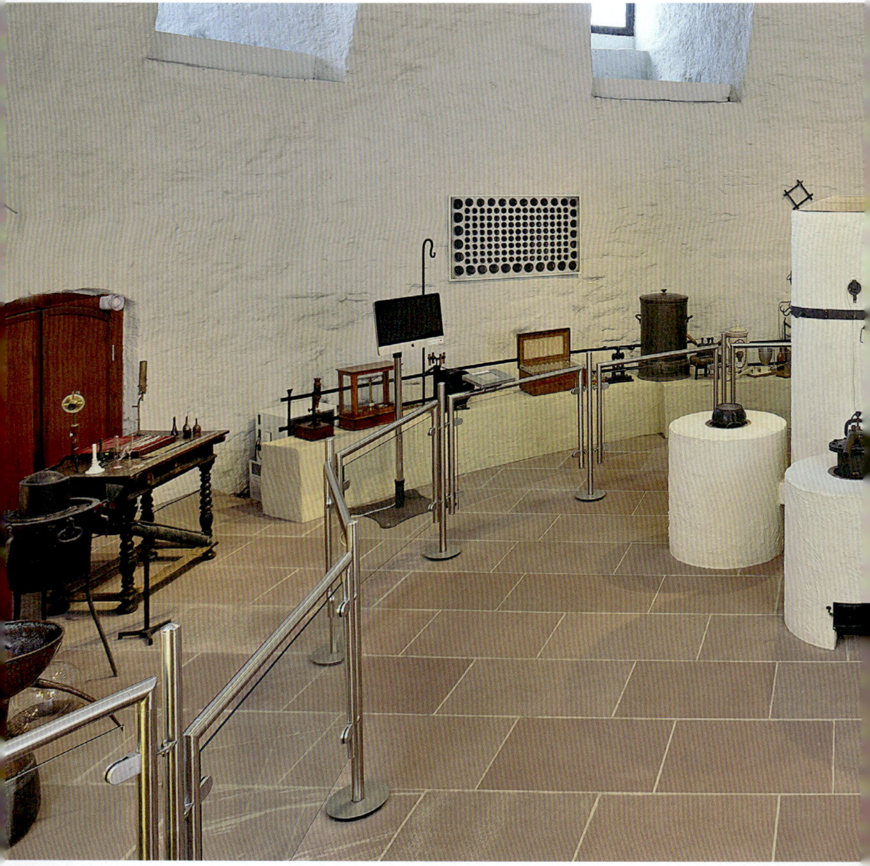

of alchemic methods. Soon, it was not possible to imagine pharmacy without distillation, for example. Essential oils and spirits (Lat. aqua vitae, the so-called water of life) became quickly famous – and not only in medicine. The installation of the laboratory equipment follows contemporary illustrations of the 16th–17th centuries, such as hearths and tools displayed in a row along the wall. In the middle of the room stands the replica of a special type of a 16th century furnace, known as "Slow Harry". Using separate channels, the main tower heats three ad-

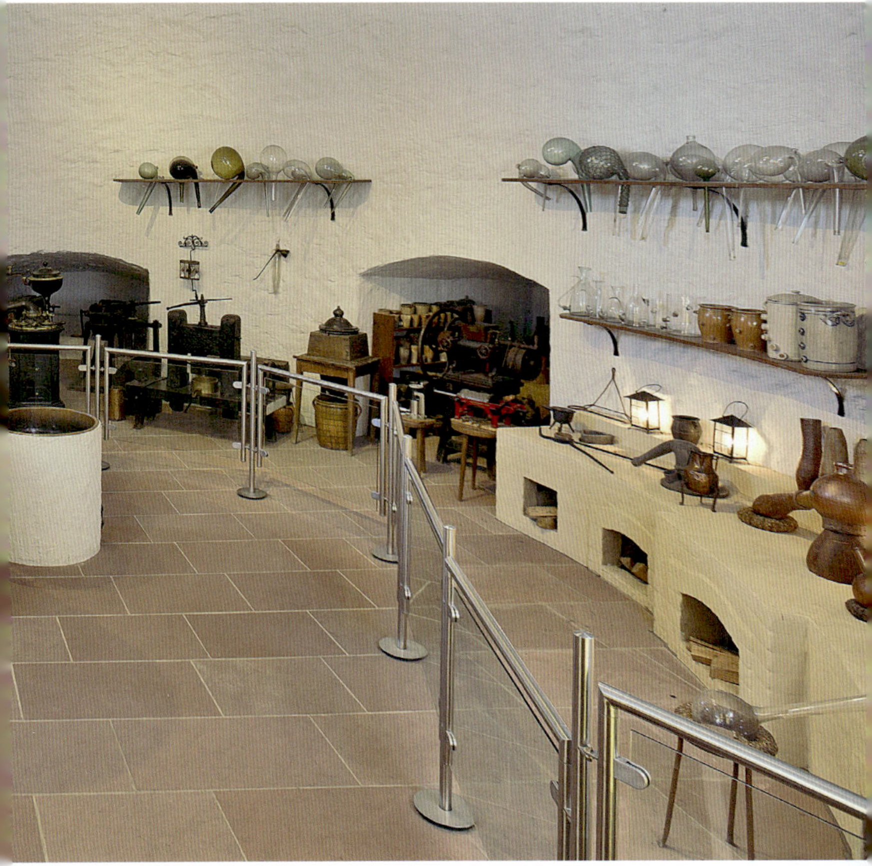

joining furnaces, which can also be used independently. Each of the four furnaces has at its disposal a grate as well as special openings for air supply. This type of furnace enabled to regulate the heat supply from the main tower to the secondary furnaces via sliding controls.

The shelves along the wall carry laboratory equipment, including a part of the worldwide largest collection of

▲ *View into the Apothecary's Tower: laboratory.*

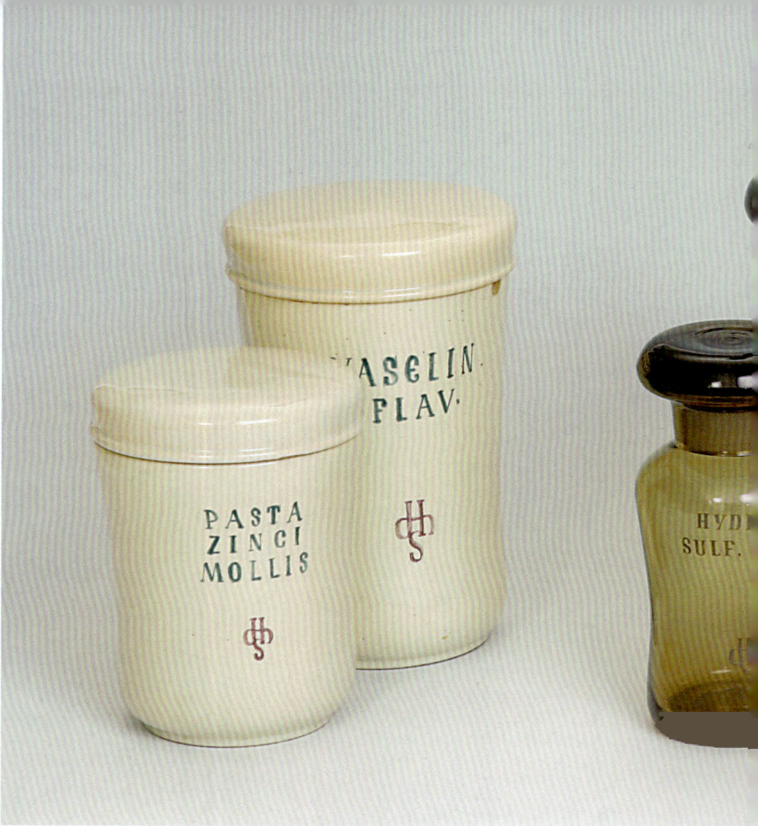

technical glasses: distillation flasks and retorts, Florentine flasks, decanters, and other typical ceramic and metal gear. Arranged according to different techniques are also diverse large-size tools, among them mighty presses like the oaken heavyweight of the Lion's Pharmacy at Landshut (17th century).

Room 11 – The Museum Shop

The furniture in the shop had originally been made for the **Diana Pharmacy at Bad Kleinen** in 1927 and today it constitutes an attractive setting for the well-stocked shop of the museum. The visitor finds here an extensive range of books, replicas of pharmaceutical vessels, confections, cosmetics, and many more articles concerning the history of pharmacy.

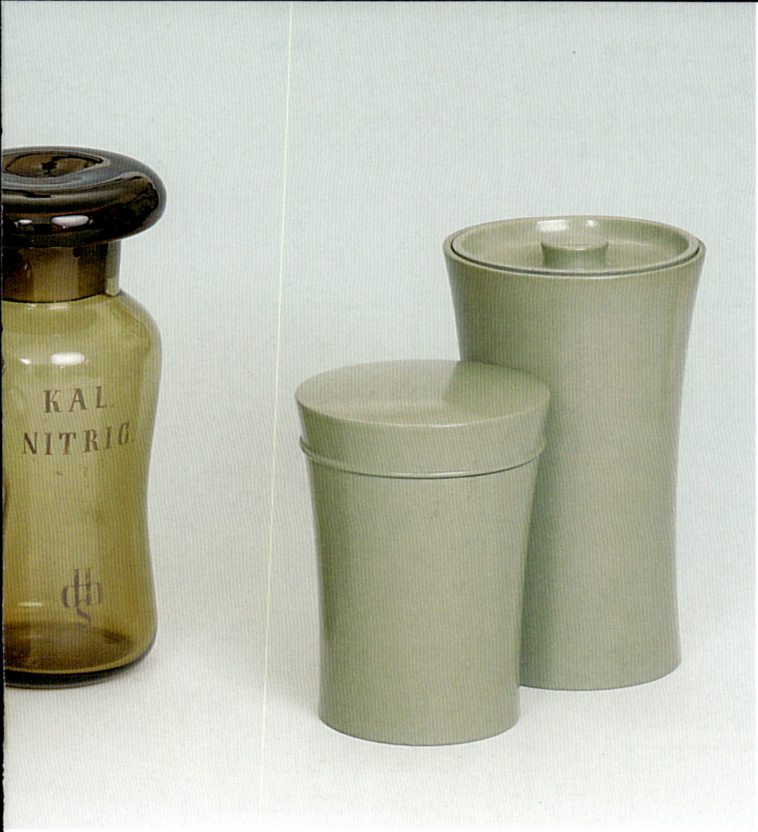

Literature

Rudolf Schmitz, Geschichte der Pharmazie, Vol. 1 – Von den Anfängen bis zum Ausgang des Mittelalters, Eschborn 1998. – Wolf-Dieter Müller-Jahncke, Christoph Friedrich – Geschichte der Pharmazie, Vol. 2 – Von der Frühen Neuzeit bis zur Gegenwart, Eschborn 2005. – Elisabeth Huwer, Das Deutsche Apotheken-Museum, Schätze aus zwei Jahrtausenden Kultur- und Pharmaziegeschichte, Regensburg 2015 (3rd edition).

▲ *Ensemble of vessels of the Sicherer Pharmacy, Heilbronn, design W. Wagenfeld/ H. Löffelhardt, 1949/50.*

Groundplan
Deutsches Apotheken-Museum

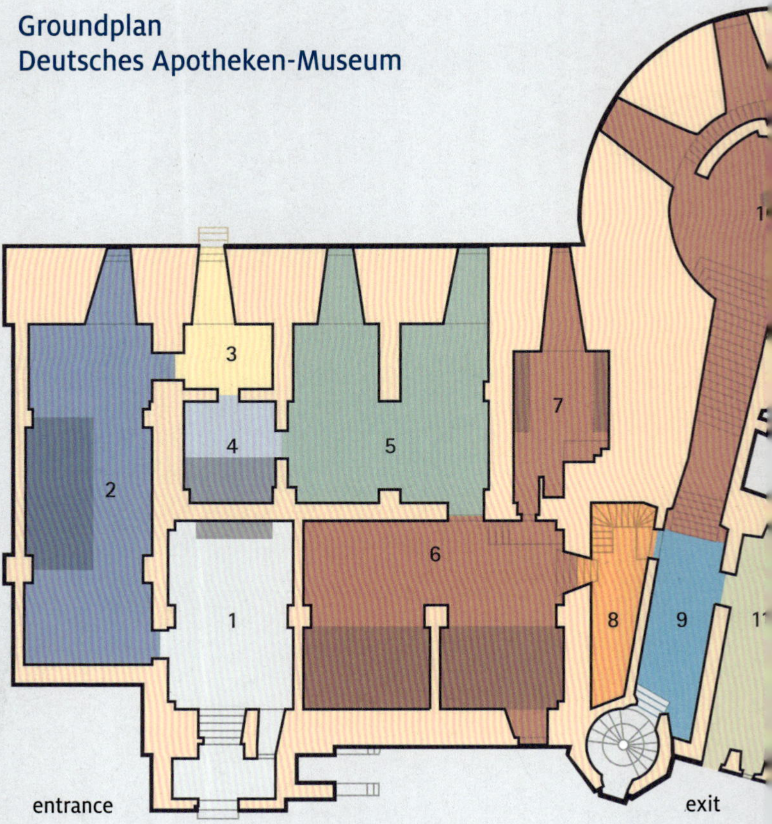

Room	**1**	Entrance / Reception
Room	**2**	Historical survey
Room	**3**	Children's pharmacy
Room	**4**	Pharmacy in the Biedermeier style
Room	**5**	The medicament
Room	**6**	The officina
Room	**7**	The store room
Room	**8**	Emblems of pharmacies
Room	**9**	Temporary exhibition
Room	**10**	The laboratory
Room	**11**	The museum shop, exit